Copyright © 20

All rights reserved. No part of this publication may be reproduced, distributed, or transmitted in any form or by any means, including photocopying, recording, or other electronic or mechanical methods, without the prior written permission of the publisher, except in the case of brief quotation embodied in critical reviews and certian other noncommercial uses permitted by copyright law.

Table of Contents

Introduction 3
What is a cannabis strain? 6
A Closer Look at Indica, Sativa, and Hybrid Strains of Marijuana
.... 10
How to choose a strain 15
Common Curiosities About Strains 17
Different types of strains 20
THC vs. CBD 27
Benefits of Cannabis 37
What are the health risks of marijuana? 66
How To Grow High Quality Cannabis (1) 69
How To Grow A Marijuana Plant From Start To Finish (2) 73
Conclusion 92

Introduction

Cannabis exists in many varieties and sub-species. Cultivators and farmers have long been breeding different varieties with certain characteristics to create hybrids and specific strains.

Each cannabis strain has a different concentration of the cannabinoids tetrahydrocannabinol (THC), cannabidiol (CBD), as well as other compounds.

Producers grow the plants to have a certain look, taste, and effect on the user and brand them accordingly.

Currently, reports on the effects of different cannabis strains come predominantly from people's experiences. Although researchers are studying the effects of a variety of cannabis strains on a range of medical conditions, there is still a long way to go in this area.

Cannabis use is on the rise in the United States. A 2018 study notes that, while cannabis use among teens has decreased, American adults are increasingly using cannabis on the daily.

According to Forbes, the global cannabis industry is estimated to be worth $7.7 billion. It's projected to hit $31.4 billion by 2021.

The industry is booming in part because cannabis can be a versatile form of medication. A number of research studies have found that cannabis has the potential to help with a variety of medical conditions, including anxiety, chronic pain, and epilepsy.

But, as any recreational or medical marijuana user can tell you, not all cannabis is created equal. Different strains of cannabis produce different effects, and thus can be used for different reasons.

You wouldn't walk into a wine shop and grab any bottle of wine thinking they were all the same. You want a wine with the flavor notes you prefer, the results you need, and the exact amount of sweetness you want. Just like that, you don't want to walk into a cannabis store and grab the first flower you see. All of those buds may appear to be similar, but their effects can be very different depending on each strain. What exactly is a cannabis strain, and why is it significant? Here is a quick guide to get you off to a good start.

What is a cannabis strain?

A strain is a genetic variation of the cannabis plant that gives the buds their aromas, effects, and appearance. Consider tomato plants as a comparison; you can have plants that produce red, yellow, orange, and even purple tomatoes. Some tomatoes will be tiny like cherries, some will be giant, and some will be pear-shaped. Tomato plants may all be tomato plants, but the fruits they bear are quite different, and even the plants themselves can have their own unique characteristics. These variances are because of differences in the plant's genetics, or the plant's strain. Cannabis plants come in many strains, each with its own unique cannabinoid production, appearance, and effects.

Just like other plants, cannabis has been cross-pollinated, genetically evolved, and even precisely bred by botanists for specific reasons. Each end result gets a new strain name like Sour Diesel, Blueberry Kush, or God's Gift because its genetics are different and its cannabinoid and terpene profile can be unique.

All strains of cannabis derive from the Cannabaceae family of plants. Some experts consider that Cannabis indica and Cannabis sativa are the two main subspecies, although some people think they are separate species.

To create a strain, cultivators select a variety of traits to produce the effects they want. This is a similar process to how breeders create particular characteristics in dogs.

People often describe cannabis strains as being indica, sativa, or hybrid. Hybrid refers to a strain created by combining both indica and sativa strains.

Strain name and Plant species

- Kush: Pure Cannabis indica or Cannabis indica hybrid
- Afghan Kush, Hindu Kush, Green Kush, Purple Kush: Pure Cannabis indica
- Blueberry Kush, Golden Jamaican Kush: Cannabis indica hybrid
- Diesel Haze: Pure Cannabis sativa or Cannabis sativa hybrid

Many producers crossbreed cannabis plants to develop new strains with specific characteristics. Experts suggest that there are over 700 strains of cannabis.

One of the most important characteristics of a cannabis strain is the THC content. Some rules exist on naming each strain, but many producers do not name their products according to these rules.

Despite these classifications, hybridization and crossbreeding has meant that people cannot tell exactly how much THC is in a particular plant by simply looking at its physical features.

Experts suggest it is impossible to guess the composition of a cannabis plant by looking at its height, branching, or leaf appearance.

The only way to know the chemical composition of a cannabis-derived product is to analyze it in a biochemical assay.

A Closer Look at Indica, Sativa, and Hybrid Strains of Marijuana

In the world of cannabis, you basically find three strain types: Indica, Sativa, and Hybrid strains. However, You do have to keep in mind that most strains have a diverse genetic background, and it can be really difficult to find a full Sativa or Indica strain. Instead, you will find that most strains are either Indica or Sativa dominant, which means the strain has more characteristics of one type or the other.

A Hybrid strain, which is obviously most prevalent, contains more balanced characteristics of both Indica or Sativa strains. Most Hybrids are created by crossing Indica-dominant and Sativa-dominant strains.

For many years, people used Indica and Sativa as a way to describe the specific effects of the strain. And, to some extent, those generalizations can be true. Therefore, we have provided some primarily experienced effects with each strain type below. Nevertheless, these experiences are not set in stone. Scientifically speaking, Sativa and Indica are used in reference to the physical traits of the plant.

Some people may use an Indica-dominant strain and be totally glued to the bed, but someone else may claim the exact same strain gave them a bit of energy. Part of this is simply due to how each individual processes cannabinoids in the plant. Further, part of the experience can be based on the specific genetics of the strain. What one grower deems Strawberry Cough, for example, may have slightly variant genetics than another grower's strain by the same name. While efforts are taken to maintain continuity in the industry, you can always find slight variations.

Take a look at a few Indica and Sativa-dominant strains, a few hybrids, and what some people experience with each.

Scout Breath cannabis flower strain
- Indica-Dominant Strains
- Death Star
- High Chew
- Salmon River OG
- Snowball
- Scout Breath
- Blue Dream
- Girl Scout Cookies

Primary Effects: Calming, Relaxing, Soothing

lemon og cannabis flower strain
- Sativa-Dominant Strains
- Lemon Brulee

- Lemon OG Haze
- Stardawg
- MTF
- Agent Orange
- Sour Diesel
- Purple Haze

Primary Effects: Energizing, Uplifting, Creative

Grape diamonds cannabis flower strain

- Hybrid Strains
- Red Dragon
- Grape Diamonds
- Apex
- NF1
- Grease Monkey
- Original Glue
- Wedding Cake

Primary Effects: Balancing, Calm but Focused, or Relaxed and Alert

How to choose a strain

The strain you choose depends on what effect you desire. As mentioned earlier, cannabis has a range of medical uses, but some strains are better for certain conditions than others.

It's also worth researching the potential adverse effects of the strain. Many of the more common strains, which you can find below, list dry mouth, dry eyes, and dizziness as possible side effects. Marijuana also has the potential to interact with medications you might be taking. Do not operate machinery when using marijuana.

Now that you have a bit of understanding of what a cannabis strain is and why it can be important to pick the right strain, how should you go about picking the best one for you? It comes down to personal preference. A few tips to remember when shopping for cannabis:

- Each strain can have characteristic flavor profiles and aromas due to terpenes
- Some strains can offer more uplifting effects, some will be more relaxing, and some offer a healthy balance
- Not every strain with the same name will deliver precisely the same effects with each use
- Do some research on each strain; Leafly gives a nice guide of many strains, and a bud-tender can always help
- Look at cannabinoid content in the strain you are considering—it does matter

Common Curiosities About Strains

What is the best cannabis strain?

"Best" can always be a matter of opinion with weed strains. Some people prefer a good couch-locked feeling while others prefer energy and focus. Each strain can yield its own unique effects, so finding the best can truly be a personal journey that has more to do with you and what you want to experience than the strain itself. If you are smoking purely for recreation, for pain relief, or something else, it is a good idea to get to know some noteworthy strains that offer aligning effects. Here are a few examples:

- Strains for Pain: Lilac Diesel, Harlequin, Jack Herer, and Agent Orange

- Strains for Sleep: Mandarin Zkittlez, Sugar Plum Sunset, 9 Pound Hammer, and Apex | Learn more
- Strains for Energy: Northern Lights, Green Crack, Red, Dragon, and Mandarin Cookies

What is the strongest strain of weed?

Cannabis strains can be dubbed as "strong" by users because they serve up some pretty impressive effects. Generally, people will refer to a strain as strong if it has a high THC content. However, the strength of the effects of a strain is not solely based on THC content. For example, if you find a strain like Cannatonic or Sour Widow, these strains can have high THC but also high CBD, which balances out the intoxicating effects of the THC. In general, Indica-dominant or hybrid plants tend to have higher amounts of CBD. Nevertheless, if you are looking for cannabis with the highest THC content, a few strains would be:

- lemon banana sherbet cannabis flower strainFire OG
- Bubba Kush
- Lemon Banana Sherbet
- Gorilla Glue
- Stardawg
- Scout Breath

How many strains of weed are there?

Some experts have claimed that about 700 unique strains of cannabis exist, but that number is an ever-growing one. New strains are born every year as botanists experiment with crossing different strains and playing around with genetics in efforts to create even more noteworthy plant qualities.

Different types of strains

According to user reviews on Leafly, here's what people might expect from a few of the most popular marijuana strains.

1. **Acapulco Gold**

   Originating from Acapulco, Mexico, Acapulco Gold is a well-known and highly praised strain of cannabis. It's noted for its euphoria-inducing, energizing effects. It's said to reduce fatigue, stress, pain, and even nausea.

2. **Blue Dream**

   Blue Dream is relaxing and soothing, but it isn't a total sedative. This makes it perfect for easing pain, cramps, or inflammation for when you can't afford to fall asleep. Plus, it's said to lift your mood and give you a feeling of euphoria.

3. **Purple Kush**

Purple Kush is great for inducing a state of bliss so that you feel relaxed, happy, and sleepy. It's often used for reducing pain and muscle spasms. Its sedating effects means it can be used to reduce insomnia.

4. **Sour Diesel**

A highly energizing, mood-lifting strain, Sour Diesel is great for giving you a burst of productive energy. It also has notable destressing and pain-relieving effects.

5. **Bubba Kush**

Bubba Kush is a relaxing, sleep-inducing strain. It's perfect for helping you fight insomnia and get some shut-eye. It also offers pain-reducing, stress-relieving results.

6. **Granddaddy Purple**

Granddaddy Purple is another highly relaxing strain. It's often praised for its insomnia-fighting and stress-reducing results. Users also note that it can make you feel euphoria and increase hunger, which is great if you're experiencing a lack of appetite.

7. **Afghan Kush**

Originating from the Hindu Kush mountains near the Afghanistan-Pakistan border, Afghan Kush is super relaxing and sleep-inducing. This, too, can help you feel hungry if you're experiencing a lack of appetite, and can relieve pain.

8. **LA Confidential**

LA Confidential is another relaxing and sleep-inducing strain that is often used to soothe insomnia. It's also said to have noticeable anti-inflammatory and pain-reducing effects, which makes it a favorite among people with chronic pain.

9. **Maui Wowie**

   Maui Wowie can help you feel super relaxed, yet energetic and creative. It reduces fatigue, too, making it great for days when you need to be productive.

10. **Golden Goat**

    Golden Goat is notable for making users feel euphoric and creative. It's also great for reducing fatigue and stress while lifting your mood.

11. **Northern Lights**

    Northern Lights is another relaxing, sleep-inducing strain. It's also known for its mood-lifting effects, and it can be used to relieve insomnia, pain, stress, and depression.

12. **White Widow**

White Widow improves your mood, gives you energy, and relaxes you all at once. It's said to help reduce pain and stress, as well as feelings of depression. If you're feeling fatigued, White Widow might help you stay energized and alert.

13. **Super Silver Haze**

Another energizing strain, Super Silver Haze is said to produce feelings of euphoria, relieves pain and nausea, and lifts your mood. This makes it excellent for stress relief.

14. **Pineapple Express**

Made famous by the 2008 eponymous movie, Pineapple Express has a pineapple-like scent. It's relaxing and mood lifting, but is also said to give you an energetic buzz. This is the sort of strain that could be great for productivity.

15. **Fruity Pebbles**

Fruity Pebbles OG, or FPOG, is associated with inducing euphoria and relaxation, which could make it great for stress relief. It often makes users feel giggly, helps reduce nausea, and increases appetite.

THC vs. CBD

So far, most research into the medical benefits of cannabis has focused on THC and CBD.

However, researchers and scientists remain unsure of the ideal quantities of THC and CBD that people should use for various medical conditions or recreation.

Although both THC and CBD are cannabinoids, they act differently in the body because they target different areas in the brain.

According to a 2020 article, people who use products with a higher THC content may experience psychoactive effects, such as euphoria and a greater sensitivity to things such as color and taste. However, THC also can lead to anxiety and paranoia.

CBD, on the other hand, is non-intoxicating. Some people report mild physiological effects, such as reduced anxiety when using CBD.

Animal studies suggest CBD may help improve vomiting, nausea, pain, and offer neuroprotective effects on the brain.

However, since CBD can affect mood, some experts describe it as a non-intoxicating but psychoactive compound.

The Food and Drug Administration (FDA) have approved some cannabis-related products including:

- two synthetic THC medications for the treatment of anorexia associated with AIDS

- another synthetic cannabis-related product for the treatment of nausea and vomiting associated with cancer treatment
- cannabis-derived CBD for children 2 years and older who suffer from rare seizure disorders

Studies are ongoing to determine whether CBD has other physiological effects. Preliminary human data suggests CBD could benefit conditions, such as schizophrenia and even opioid addiction.

Sativa vs. Indica

The terms indica and sativa derive from the biolgical classification of these species, which is based on physical characteristics. Cannabis indica plants are shorter and have broad, dark green leaves. Cannabis sativa plants grow taller and develop thinner, pale green leaves.

In the past, people used these terms to differentiate the cannabis plants in terms of their effects and THC or CBD content. An article in Cannabis and Cannabinoid Research seems to dispel these claims.

Previously, people believed that Cannabis indica plants contained higher levels of CBD. As a result, cultivators and dispensaries marketed indica-derived strains as a product that would lead to a more 'relaxed high'.

Conversely, Cannabis sativa-derived strains that contained higher levels of THC would provide a more energetic high.

Many experts caution against this generalization, noting that even if this classification scheme were true, there is no way to be sure of the accuracy of any strain name.

There is no third-party agency that validates which strain names belong to indica, sativa, or hybrid.

To know exactly what is in a cannabis product, the manufacturers must analyze the product in a biochemical assay.

It is easy to see why this topic continues to cause debate. Cannabis is a complex plant, and, as of right now, there seems no obvious or simple way to categorize the various strains by 'effect on the user.'

Each person who tries a strain of cannabis may have a different experience.

For example, some people describe the effects of Cannabis indica-derived products as sedating. However, other components of cannabis can also cause sedation, as well as other psychoactive effects. Compounds include:

- linalool
- myrcene
- limonene
- alpha-pinene

These components are often absent in a description of a cannabis-derived product, which is why some experts suggest that manufacturers should abandon naming their products as sativa or indica. Using these names is misleading and far more complex than people once thought.

Useful products

If marijuana is legal in your state and you're interested in trying — or even growing — different types of cannabis strains, there are a number of products that can make your life a little easier.

Volcano Vaporizer

Some people might prefer inhaling cannabis over smoking it through a pipe, bong, or joint. This desktop vaporizer heats up cannabis and expels the vapor into a balloon. The person then inhales the air from the balloon.

The vaporizer can be used with dried herbs or liquid concentrates, and can be purchased here.

Magical Butter Kit

Cannabutter — or cannabis-infused butter — is the basis of many edibles. Unfortunately, making cannabutter can be a lengthy and labor-intensive process.

This butter kit, however, makes it easy to infuse herbs into butter. It has its own heating unit and thermostat, which ensures that the product and butter are at the ideal temperature throughout the process.

tCheck Dosage Checker

The tCheck Dosage Checker tests the strength of cannabis-infused liquids — like alcohol-based tinctures. It can also test cannabis-infused olive oil, ghee (clarified butter), and coconut butter, which will help you determine how strong your edibles are before you indulge.

Unfortunately, it only checks liquids, not dried herb.

Palm Mincer

Grinding up cannabis can be time-consuming, so the Palm Mincer can be quite useful. It fits perfectly into your palm, and it can be used to chop up cannabis quickly and efficiently. What's more it's dishwasher safe, so it's easy to clean off the sticky cannabis resin. You can buy it I here.

Harvest Starter Kit

If you want to start growing your own cannabis, this convenient starter kit contains everything you need to harvest it.

The grow kit includes a trimming tray, a microscope for examining the buds to determine whether they're ready for harvest, three types of pruning shears, a disinfecting spray for your tools, a drying rack, and gloves.

Note: Even if marijuana is legal in your state, it continues to be illegal under federal law.

Benefits of Cannabis

1. **It May Aid In Weight Loss**

   The age-old stereotype of the "stoner" is typically accompanied by two key characteristics: laziness and an insatiable bout of the munchies. While certain strains of cannabis show evidence of causing consumers to take in more calories, further research suggests that regular cannabis users tend to have a lower Body Mass Index than the average person who does not use cannabis. This is because of the plant's ability to regulate insulin production and overall caloric effect.

2. **It May Regulate and/or Prevent Diabetes**

Keeping in mind that cannabis helps regulate insulin production and control weight, it makes sense why some could see its potential to help patients with diabetes. Consequently, a 2013 study revealed the following: cannabis compounds may play a role in controlling blood sugar, lowering BMI, and increasing levels of "good cholesterol." Additionally, a 2015 study on the effects of cannabidiol (CBD) suggests that the cannabinoid's anti-inflammatory properties may work as an effective treatment for Type 2 diabetes.

3. **It May Help Fight Cancer**

While medical cannabis has been used by patients enduring chemotherapy to soothe the intense side effects, recent research suggests that cannabis may be able to inhibit and/or kill cancer cells without affecting normal white blood cells. Researchers believe that cannabis with higher amounts of CBD (or pure CBD isolate) may be even more effective in killing cancer cells, which could be groundbreaking for the medical community if further tested or elaborated on.

4. **It May Ease Symptoms Of Depression**

As depression and anxiety become increasingly common in today's society, so does the need for relief. From oral medication to therapies, there are several treatments available for depression, and cannabis may be one of them. Researchers at the University of Buffalo have been studying the link between cannabis and depression. Their findings have revealed that depressed people tend to have reduced endocannabinoid levels, which could be resolved by using cannabis to restore the system's balance.

5. **It Has Shown Promise In Treating Autism**

For those living with Autism Spectrum Disorder, cannabis may be an effective treatment for symptoms, without the significant side effects some experience from the two FDA-approved psychotics. Cannabis, specifically CBD, helps regulate mood, which could be helpful with the social and cognitive struggles that people with autism may experience. Some parents of autistic children have begun to use CBD and THCA oil to help regulate mood swings and other challenging symptoms.

6. **It May Protect you From Coronavirus**

While there is still very little known about COVID-19 and how it is prevented and/or treated, there seems to be evidence that suggests cannabis may help. Researchers are looking into whether the plant may reduce coronavirus susceptibility as well as its potential to stop deadly cytokine storms.

7. **It Helps Regulate Seizures**

Medical cannabis has been used to treat a variety of ailments over the years, including seizures and epilepsy in children and adults. EPIDIOLEX, the first prescription, plant-derived cannabinoid medicine in the U.S., is an FDA-approved formulation of highly purified cannabidiol (CBD) used specifically for the treatment of seizures and epilepsy.

8. **It May Decrease Healing Time In Broken Bones**

If you've ever broken a bone before, you're well aware how agonizing the recovery process can feel. Researchers have discovered that cannabis, specifically CBD, seems to enhance the healing process in fractured bones. A study done by the American Society for Bone and Mineral Research found the healing process in rats with broken leg bones was drastically improved after just eight weeks.

9. **It Has Shown Promise In Easing ADHD Symptoms**

For those who have trouble concentrating or suffer from ADD or ADHD, cannabis may be an effective solution. While medication exists like Ritalin or Adderall, cannabis might be a safer alternative with a lower risk of unwanted side effects. Patients who've used cannabis to self-treat their symptoms have reported the plant may help with agitation, irritability, and lack of restraint.

10. **It May Aid In Serious Addiction Recovery**

Cannabis may work as an aid in addiction recovery. In the midst of our country's opioid crisis, patients have reported the plant's ability to help soothe the withdrawal symptoms that come with detoxing from drugs like heroin or other opiates. And states with medical marijuana laws saw a 20 percent drop in some opioid prescriptions.

11. **It May Treat Glaucoma**

Ever since we first began to see medical cannabis legalization throughout the country, glaucoma was a popular reason for patients to apply for their medical cards. As the leading cause of blindness in the world, glaucoma is not an ailment to be ignored. Cannabis use seems to reduce intraocular pressure, which is a key contributor to the disease.

12. **It May Improve Lung Health**

This may seem counterintuitive, especially since the act of smoking has quite a stigma when it comes to lung health, but researchers believe ingesting cannabis does not have any adverse effects on the lungs — in fact, it may improve lung health. If you're still worried, opt out of smoking and try edibles or tinctures as an alternative — all the benefit of the plant without the toxins associated with smoking.

13. **It Shows Promise In Easing Anxiety**

But be careful — while cannabis may cause anxiety in some users, it can decrease anxiety in others. However, this is more specific to tetrahydrocannabinol (THC), the cannabinoid responsible for the "high" effect of cannabis.

CBD seems to have a better track record when it comes to curbing anxiety.

14. **It May Slow The Development of Alzheimer's Disease**

Recent studies have suggested that cannabis may possess the ability to slow the progress of Alzheimer's disease, which would be groundbreaking for the elderly community.

15. **It May Help Patients With Multiple Sclerosis**

For patients suffering from Multiple Sclerosis, it can be difficult to find an effective treatment for controlling muscle spasms. Cannabis may help soothe the pain and reduce the intake of prescription drugs that may have a long list of side effects.

16. **It May Calm & Control Muscle Spasms**

    As patients with M.S. discover cannabis as a possible solution for their muscle spasms, it becomes applicable to anyone who suffers from muscle spasms unrelated to M.S. Researchers have found that cannabis tends to decrease muscle spasms in patients who struggle with stiff, aching, cramping muscles.

17. **It May Help Eating Disorder Recovery Progress**

    While many believe eating disorders to be physical illnesses, they are actually mental illnesses with extreme physical side effects. Evidence suggests that sufferers may have a chemical imbalance directly related to the endocannabinoid system, and cannabis use may help bring order to this imbalance and regulate appetite.

18. **It Has Been Used To Treat Arthritis**

Among the increasing number of ailments it's being used to treat, CBD may have a positive effect on patients suffering from arthritis. Animal studies have suggested that CBD's pain-relieving, anti-inflammatory properties may ease the effects of arthritis.

19. **It May Ease PTSD Symptoms**

From war veterans to sexual assault survivors, PTSD is an illness that afflicts many. Luckily, cannabis seems to be an effective treatment for the harrowing symptoms, regulating mood, and overall anxiety and panic.

20. **It May Help Regulate Metabolism**

In the same vein that cannabis may help patients lose weight, the plant may also help to regulate metabolism. Its effect on insulin and other metabolic hormones suggests it may play a role in helping those who have metabolic issues.

21. **It Can Help Ease Medication Side Effects For Those With AIDS/HIV**

While cannabis cannot directly cure AIDS/HIV, it has been a recognized treatment for the adverse side effects of medications used to treat the disease since its initial outbreak in the 1980s. In fact, Michael Koehn's lobbying for medical cannabis as a treatment for those with

AIDS/HIV was the reason California first legalized medical cannabis in 1996.

22. It May Be Effective For Treating Nausea

There are several causes for nausea and/or vomiting, but not too many solutions. However, considerable evidence suggests that regulating the endocannabinoid system with cannabis use may in turn regulate nausea.

23. It May Soothe Headaches

According to recent studies, cannabis seems to decrease headache and migraine severity by nearly 50%. This would be an ideal alternative to prescription drugs or pills that can have unsavory side effects.

24. **It May Treat Acne**

Acne is a common and often difficult skin condition to address, but research suggests that cannabis could offer a path to relief. While more research is needed, a study published in the Journal of Clinical Investigation found that CBD inhibited oil production and also had anti-inflammatory effects on oil-producing glands.

25. **It May Help Speech Problems**

From stuttering to other voice disorders, speech disorders can be frustrating to work through. Depending on the cause of the speech disorder, cannabis may work as an effective treatment for any spasms or twitches that may accompany the issue.

26. **It May Improve Skin Conditions**

Cannabis isn't just for smoking — with the emergence of cannabis topicals and creams, people are beginning to use the plant to rub on pains, aches, and even skin conditions like skin cancer, eczema, or psoriasis.

27. **It May Soothe Chemotherapy Side Effects**

As mentioned earlier, cannabis has been used by patients with cancer to better endure the difficult side effects, especially from the effects of chemotherapy. Patients who undergo chemotherapy usually experience intense nausea, and the plant has a track record that suggests it may be a useful treatment.

28. **It May Regulate Obsessive Compulsive Disorder**

While anxiety and stress can be heightened in some people who use cannabis, CBD has reportedly worked well to soothe these symptoms. Similarly, it may help those with Obsessive Compulsive Disorder (OCD). A study done on rats revealed that, even at low doses, CBD was able to reverse OCD symptoms.

29. **It May Calm Asthma Attacks**

Since cannabis has shown signs of being able to improve lung health, it makes sense to assume it may also be able to soothe those with asthma. However, proceed with caution: smoking cannabis may drastically worsen asthmatic symptoms, but ingesting cannabinoids in tincture or edible form may help ease symptoms.

30. **It May Be A Natural Alternative To Viagra**

From headaches to nausea to overall pain, there are several risky side effects that come with taking Viagra. However, cannabis has been used as an aphrodisiac for centuries and may be a natural solution to popping pills.

31. **It May Help Lower Blood Pressure**

Another possible benefit of using cannabis is that it may help lower your blood pressure. In a study where healthy volunteers were given a single dose of CBD, the blood pressure in all subjects was reduced, which suggests that regular usage may result in an overall lower blood pressure.

32. It May Soothe Panic Attacks

As previously mentioned, cannabis (and specifically CBD) have been reported to work as an anxiety regulator, although this can depend on the strain, the dosage, and the person. Keeping that in mind, studies have found that cannabis may soothe panic attack symptoms for those who suffer.

33. It Can Be Used As A Food Source

Although cannabis isn't lining the shelves at our grocery stores today, the plant has been used as a food source by several communities throughout history. Hemp has been used as a valuable protein source, and is even found as an ingredient in protein powders today.

34. It's A Great Investment Opportunity

With the increase of states offering legal adult-use and/or medical cannabis, the industry is booming more and more every day. And with even more states adding legal cannabis to their ballots for November, now is the time to invest.

35. It May Help Fight Climate Change

As the cannabis market begins to legalize throughout the nation, we'll see an increase in large-scale cannabis farms, which could have an overall positive effect on the environment. Experts say it may help reduce CO_2 emissions, which may help reverse the effects of climate change over time.

36. **The Cannabis Industry Creates Jobs**

Along with valuable investment opportunities, the increase of legal cannabis has allowed for a massive amount of job creation. From growers to doctors to budtenders, the growing industry has endless opportunities for a good paycheck.

37. **Cannabis Generates Revenue For Public Programs**

Another benefit of legalizing cannabis is the revenue the states get to enjoy from the sales taxes. In states where cannabis is legal, they're seeing a large amount of revenue from cannabis sales, which are then funneled into public programs like schools, health programs, cannabis research, and more.

38. **Legal Cannabis Will Clean Up People's Records**

As states are working to legalize cannabis, they are also working to expunge records of those who were wrongfully locked up for trivial cannabis charges over the past several decades. The MORE Act, which will be voted on by the House this year, will work to decriminalize cannabis on a federal level and expunge some criminal records.

39. **Legal Cannabis Creates New Industries**

In tandem with the job creation that cannabis allows for, it's also created new opportunities for existing industries. According to experts, the cannabis industry is the fastest growing industry in the U.S. today, and allows for industries like medicine, beauty, banking, agriculture, advertising, food, and more to get involved.

40. **Legal Cannabis May Lower Crime Rates**

As cannabis continues to remove its prohibited status, the states will continue to see a dip in crime rates. This is a pretty obvious result of legalizing something that was previously illegal, but states that have legalized cannabis have seen overall drops in crime, including violent crimes unrelated to cannabis.

41. **Legal Cannabis May Lead To Safer Roads**

An economics study revealed that, in states where cannabis has been legalized, they've seen a drop in traffic deaths. There has coincidentally been a sizable drop in alcohol sales in legal states, which may contribute to the drop in traffic deaths.

42. Legal Cannabis Cheapens Law Enforcement Costs

In Colorado, a state that has offered legal adult-use cannabis since 2012, there has been a drop in taxpayer costs due to the fact that law enforcement is no longer spending money on cannabis arrests. This also frees up law enforcements' time and allows for them to focus on real crime.

43. **It May Help Keep Your Pets Healthy**

As CBD continues to flood the cannabis market with its non-psychoactive healing properties, we're seeing that it works for all sorts of people, from children to adults — and now, even pets. For animals who are sick, living with chronic pain, or suffering from anxiety or depression, cannabis may be a viable natural treatment.

44. **It May Improve Your Dreams**

If you suffer from PTSD or other mental disorders, you may also be plagued with endless nightmares that leave you more exhausted when you wake up than when you went to sleep. Luckily, CBD and THC both seem to have an effect on your REM cycle, which can allow for more pleasant dreams, or the inability to remember your nightmares.

45. It May Increase Energy Levels

Proceed with caution, as this can vary greatly depending on the strain and your body/mind, but certain strains of cannabis may work to boost your energy levels. Keep an eye out for strains that contain terpenes like pinene and limonene, which tend to have more uplifting effects.

46. It May Help Improve Sleep

Conversely, other strains of cannabis may help improve your sleep and fight insomnia. Researchers have found that cannabis may help regulate your sleep cycle overall, specifically in strains that have higher levels of THC than CBD.

47. **It May Improve Your Work Day**

Depending on what you do for a living, cannabis may help improve your workday. It isn't necessarily recommended to smoke a bunch before you go in for the day, especially if you have a high-stress, high-engagement role, but there are several CBD options for regulating your mood without having any psychoactive effects that may negatively impact your productivity.

48. **It May Improve Your Digestive System**

Whether you suffer from digestive issues like Irritable Bowel Syndrome or gastritis, cannabis may work as a reliever. As most digestive issues are a result of inflammation, the anti-inflammatory effects of cannabis (and specifically CBD) may play a role in healing.

49. **It May Boost Creativity**

As with productivity levels, this will depend on the strain, the dosage, and the person, but cannabis seems to have an overall positive effect on creativity. More studies need to be done to confirm exactly how cannabis should be used to boost creativity, but it seems that a cannabis-induced state of mind tends to allow for more divergent thinking in consumers.

50. It May Protect Your Brain

We mentioned earlier that cannabis may have positive effects on reversing the progression of Alzheimer's disease, and studies have found that cannabis seems to have an overall positive neurological effect on consumers. Cannabinoids like CBD and THC have neuroprotective effects, which may work to protect and preserve our brain cells.

What are the health risks of marijuana?

At the other end of the spectrum is the plethora of studies that have found negative associations between marijuana use and health. They are listed below.

1. **Mental health problems**

    Daily marijuana use is believed to exacerbate existing symptoms of bipolar disorder among people who have this mental health problem. However, the National Academies of Sciences, Engineering, and Medicine report suggests that among people with no history of the condition, there is only limited evidence of a link between marijuana use and developing bipolar disorder.

    Moderate evidence suggests that regular marijuana users are more likely to experience suicidal thoughts, and there is a small increased risk of depression among marijuana users.

Marijuana use is likely to increase risk of psychosis, including schizophrenia. But a curious finding among people with schizophrenia and other psychoses is that a history of marijuana use is linked with improved performance on tests assessing learning and memory.

2. **Testicular cancer**

Although there is no evidence to suggest any link between using marijuana and an increased risk for most cancers, the National Academies of Sciences did find some evidence to suggest an increased risk for the slow-growing seminoma subtype of testicular cancer.

3. Respiratory disease

Regular marijuana smoking is linked to increased risk of chronic cough, but "it is unclear" whether smoking marijuana worsens lung function or increases the risk of chronic obstructive pulmonary disease or asthma.

A 2014 study that explored the relationship between marijuana use and lung disease suggested that it was plausible that smoking marijuana could contribute to lung cancer, though it has been difficult to conclusively link the two.

How To Grow High Quality Cannabis (1)

Being able to produce cannabis on your own is one thing, but knowing how to grow high-quality cannabis is another. With more states legalizing marijuana use, you want to make sure you're getting the highest quality buds. While achieving this can be challenging even for seasoned growers, our growing marijuana 101 can help you realize your goal. Read on to learn how to grow a marijuana plant from start to finish, including the secrets behind producing premium cannabis buds!

1. **Pick Reliable Cannabis Seed Banks**

   When purchasing cannabis seeds, you might often choose the cheapest ones to save some bucks. However, the quality may be compromised, and you'll end up spending more than you have to. That's why you should pick cannabis seeds with the best genetics. Conduct your research so that you can buy from trusted cannabis seed banks. Cloning can be a good start too — just make sure to get the clones from reputable sources.

2. **Provide Enough Lighting**

One essential element for growing cannabis is proper lighting. It's not only the quality that will be affected but also the speed and size. While marijuana grown outdoors gets natural light, indoor cannabis needs extra care. This means that your usual lightbulbs are not enough to make up for the absence of lights.

Invest in more premium lights, hoods, and reflectors. Get high-intensity (HID) lights, like high-pressure sodium (HPS) or T5 fluorescent lights. You can also use LEDs to save on energy costs. Just make sure to choose full-spectrum LED lights that allow you to modify the wavelength based on the marijuana plant's needs as it grows.

3. **Enhance Water Quality**

Dissolved solids from water can cause adverse effects on your marijuana plant. For instance, domestic water contains chlorine and fluoride. While they will not kill the plant, maximum yield can't be expected. So, consider using a reverse osmosis system or filtration. Make sure to change the filters regularly. It's also best to test the water from time to time to check whether the parts per million (PPM) of dissolved solids remain the same.

4. **Secure Enough Spacing And Ventilation**

Wondering how to grow high-quality marijuana? Allow enough spacing between the cannabis buds. Make sure no leaves or branches block the airflow. You can apply low stress training (LST) where you tie the plants down while they're still young to ensure that the light is well-dispersed, improving the plant's overall health. Using other tools like filters and fans will also help you maintain the airflow.

How To Grow A Marijuana Plant From Start To Finish (2)

1. **Provide Sufficient Amount Of Nutrients**

One of the 10 steps to growing weed is providing just the right amount of nutrients per growth stage.

Tribus Original is the perfect seedling to harvest cannabis growing products on the market today and it's very versatile. Usage rates are 1 ml per gallon and with a price tag under $60 for a 250 ml bottle, and a little goes a long way. Because it consists of beneficial bacteria you really can't overfeed your cannabis plants with it, and it creates stronger plants from the inside out. For best results apply it to your grow media at least once a week. Tribus is compatible with all grow media, including hydroponics and even field application.

In addition to Tribus, these nutrients are necessary when feeding cannabis plants.

- Nitrogen: In the vegetative stage, marijuana plants will need an abundant amount of nitrogen. However, in the flowering stage, it has to be reduced. Otherwise, it can affect the production of buds and lead to lower yields. Biostimulants and different types of soil amendments can help plants absorb more nutrients. The best soil amendments that enhance nitrogen include Guano, worm castings, and crustacean meal.
- Potassium: A sufficient amount of potassium in the flowering stage helps promote the plant's health and growth. If it's lacking, the growth

rate will decline, causing problems for the leaves. Natural soil amendments for potassium include wood ash, compost, and seaweed meal.

- Phosphorus: When there's a phosphorus deficiency, smaller leaves dry fast and turn purplish with seared edges. That is why the plants should be rich in phosphorus during the flowering stage. Dry soil amendments for phosphorus are glacial rock dust, chicken manure, and bone meal. Pick trusted soil amendment suppliers to achieve the best results.
- Nitrogen, potassium, and phosphorus may be the three main nutrients that your cannabis plants need. However, they also need other nutrients like:

- Magnesium: This nutrient is crucial in photosynthesis. It helps stabilize plant cell walls too.
- Calcium: This micronutrient helps strengthen the stems, form the roots, and facilitate the growth of the tips. If calcium is lacking, tips become weak, and leaves get distorted.
- Sulfur: Your plant should have the right amount of sulfur to form chlorophyll and help produce amino acids, vitamins, and enzymes. Inadequacy can make the marijuana leaves stiff and small, hampering their growth. Then, they will die off.
- Manganese: If your cannabis plant lacks manganese, the leaves will turn yellow with white, gray, or brown spots. These will soon spread, causing the leaves to die.

During the flowering stage, various supplements can be beneficial too. These include:

- Phosphorus and Potassium boosters: These supplements contain Phosphorus and Potassium, but they may also include a little bit of sulfur. Trace minerals, amino acids, and sugar may also be present. As they are potent enough, use a small amount only.
- Carbohydrates or sugar: These help enhance the plant's smell and taste. Other supplements also come with specific terpenes that contribute to buds' flavors, such as berry and citrus. If you prefer a more affordable choice, you can use blackstrap molasses to add sugar and amino acids. They can enhance your plant's taste and smell when you give them several weeks before harvest time.

- Bloom enhancers: These help increase plant growth rate by supplying amino acids and humic acids. This way, the marijuana plant won't have to produce everything on its own.

2. **Prune Cannabis Properly**

While low stress training does not involve cutting, you have to perform pruning to promote yield increase in plants. It also helps you get rid of buds that are not in their best condition. This way, buds become fewer but larger and healthier. Consider removing the lowest branches to ward off pests. To ensure that the plants recover and grow faster, prune during the vegetation stage.

3. **Keep The Right Room Temperature And Humidity**

Cannabis can grow well under several conditions, but you need to ensure that the room's temperature and humidity satisfy the weed's needs. Even small changes can affect its growth, so focus on the temperature and humidity in each stage.

4. **Seedling Stage**

For seedlings and clones, the preferred humidity levels range from 65% to 80%. This way, they can take up enough water and have stronger roots. In terms of temperature, keep it at 25 degrees Celsius or 77 degrees Fahrenheit during the day and 21 degrees Celsius or 70 degrees Fahrenheit during the night.

5. **Vegetative Stage**

   In the vegetative stage, moderate humidity levels are necessary. Every week, you can decrease it by 5%. Around 40% to 70% will work. Given that the roots are stronger during this period, they can absorb more water, so lowered humidity levels are preferred. For the temperature, you can raise it a bit — around 71 to 82 degrees Fahrenheit during the day and around 64 degrees Fahrenheit to 75 degrees Fahrenheit at night.

6. **Flowering Stage**

   Reducing the humidity levels to 40% to 50% is needed during the flowering stage. You can make it 55% but never 60%. Also, the temperature can decrease to 68 to 78 degrees

Fahrenheit. Then, in the latter part of the flowering period or one to two weeks prior to harvest, reduce humidity levels from 30% to 40%.

Meanwhile, the temperature can fall between 64 to 75 degrees Fahrenheit or 18 to 24 degrees Celsius with lights on and 16 to 20 degrees Celsius for several nights before harvest. To monitor the humidity and temperature, use a hygrometer and thermometer.

7. **Lowering Temperature**

If you aim to lower the temperature, you can do the following:
- During the day, keep the lights off; during the night, on.

- Add an air conditioning unit. This can also help reduce humidity.
- Use a cool tube if you are growing marijuana with HPS lights.

8. **Increasing Temperature**

    To raise the temperature, you can:

- Utilize a quality space heater with a thermostat.
- Use grow lights with higher watts.
- At the bottom of your grow room or tent, place a heating mat.

9. **Lowering Humidity**

    If you want to drop the humidity levels, perform these steps:

- Water your marijuana plants immediately after switching on the lights. Given the quick absorption, humidity levels will decrease.
- Get a humidifier.
- Have an airflow fan upgrade to increase the supply of cool air.

10. **Increasing Humidity**

Enhancing humidity levels can be possible through the following:

- Use a humidifier that has enough water reservoir to avoid frequent refills.
- Using a spray bottle, mist your marijuana plants. However, this shouldn't be done to flowering plants as it can result in bud rot.

- Bring larger plants inside the room. Compared to seedlings, they perspire more, raising the humidity levels in the grow room.
- Consider hanging wet towels inside your grow room.

11. **Maintain Enough Co2**

Did you know that providing your marijuana plants with sufficient carbon dioxide (co2) helps improve their growth by 20%? Co2 is crucial in photosynthesis, where cannabis absorbs light and turns it into energy. Excessive co2 or a lack of it can be detrimental to your cannabis plants. So, you should know how to provide them with the right co2 levels. Ideally, it should be above 250 ppm.

To supplement your plants with extra CO_2, you can use the following:

- CO_2 generator: To produce carbon dioxide, the CO_2 generator burns natural gas or propane. It automatically turns on or off if a certain CO_2 level is reached. However, burning the gasses can create heat. So, it's advisable to use one in a larger grow room.
- Compressed CO_2: With this option, the manufacturer produces the gas and compresses it into a tank. No heat is produced once gasses are released, so you won't have issues with the temperature and humidity levels. It can also be set to automatic using a controller. Note, however, that both CO_2 generators and compressed CO_2 can be relatively costly.
- CO_2 bags: To produce carbon dioxide, these utilize fungi from organic matter. However,

even if you have a small grow room, you need four or more CO2 bags. This way, you can get the desired PPM.

- Dry ice: Cold and solid carbon dioxide comprises dry ice. Once it warms up, it releases carbon dioxide into the air. It's an effective short-term solution, but given its price, if used in the long term, it's not practical. Also, you need to constantly add dry ice daily. It's hard to control the amount of carbon dioxide in the air, too.
- Fermentation: This process produces carbon dioxide naturally. However, it should be noted that significantly less CO2 is produced. Also, fermentation comes with an unwanted odor.
- Compost: This produces a relatively small CO2 amount. Aside from it being unhygienic, you don't know whether you're adding an adequate amount of carbon dioxide.

12. Know When To Harvest The Cannabis Plants

Harvest time keeps growers excited, especially given all the efforts exerted to produce healthy and quality buds. However, cutting them too soon will defeat the purpose and waste all your hard work as the tetrahydrocannabinol (THC) content will be low. So, harvest them at the right time based on the following indications:

- Trichome color: Trichomes refer to the appendages on the cannabis flower's surface. They're the ones that hold the plant's natural compounds, like THC and terpenes. If half of them appear milky white, and the other half become amber, it's a good sign to harvest. However, if most of them are clear, that means the plants are not yet ready for harvest. As it's a bit challenging to see the color of the trichomes, you might want to use a magnifying glass.

- Brown pistils: Another way to tell the right time to harvest is through the pistils. When they mature, they turn brown. Using a magnifying glass to check the color is also recommended here.
- Bud shape: Unlike the trichome color test, this one's not a definite way to tell whether your plant should be harvested. However, it helps you determine whether the plant has matured. Aside from the shape, check whether the buds are firm and tight.
- Curling leaves: One common sign to harvest is when the leaves curl and dry. This is expected because when it's almost harvest time, the plants will absorb less water.
- Leaf color: While the leaves turn green during the flowering phase, they become yellow when

it's about time to harvest them. Given that nitrogen is reduced, the leaves also start falling off.

13. **Dry And Cure Cannabis Properly**

You may think you're done once you harvest your cannabis. However, drying and curing are important steps to producing quality and tasty buds. First, drying helps reduce the bud's moisture content to 15%. It also enables you to maintain its taste and the natural compounds in it, including THC. To dry cannabis properly, follow these steps:

- Cut down your cannabis plants. While most growers prefer to cut off the branches, some want to cut until the base and hang them upside down. Others will also cut off each bud and then place them on a drying rack.

- Trim to remove larger fan leaves. Doing so will contribute to your buds' improved look. If you're residing in a place with less than 30% humidity levels, trim fewer leaves.
- Begin the slow drying process. A temperature of 65 to 75 degrees Fahrenheit and 50% humidity is preferred. If it exceeds 80 degrees, the terpene content will go away. While hanging the buds upside down is the most common method, you can use a drying rack or cardboard to lay them out. Generally, you need three to seven days to dry the buds well.

After the drying process, you can now proceed to curing to preserve the plant's cannabinoids or compounds and terpenes. Simply perform the following:

- Put the cannabis buds into mason jars with a wide opening. Other alternatives include plastic or wooden vessels.
- Secure the container in a dark and dry area. Humidity levels should range from 60% to 65%.
- Check the containers regularly. Open them at least once a day for two weeks. Doing so will remove extra moisture and accommodate fresh air.
- While your cannabis should be ready for use in two to three weeks, keeping it for around two months is recommended for maximum results. Commercial grow operations may prefer to use chemicals to hasten production. However, the whole experience of users may be compromised.

Conclusion

Since cannabis is more readily available today than ever before, people need clear, accurate information on the effects of different cannabis strains for medical and recreational purposes.

Knowing the composition and physiological and mental effects of cannabis plants can help people and clinicians choose the most appropriate product.

Cannabis farmers crossbreed cannabis plants to create new strains that have different levels of THC, CBD, and many other physiologically active compounds.

Each plant may have different medicinal and recreational purposes. Researchers need to carry out further studies to better understand this complex plant and its effects on humans.

Marijuana can be beneficial to a variety of individuals, especially those living with certain conditions causing pain, intense vomiting, or severe lack of appetite. Like many medications or supplements, weed might have the potential to become addictive in some individuals.

Addiction involves a number of factors, and the lack of clear statistics on weed makes this a complicated topic. If you're worried about the potential for addiction, talk with your doctor about your concerns.

Made in the USA
Monee, IL
26 September 2022

14686416R00056